CulturalCare

Guides to Heritage Assessment and HEALTH Traditions

**RACHEL E. SPECTOR, PH.D.,
R.N., C.T.N., F.A.A.N.**

Prentice Hall Health
Upper Saddle River, New Jersey 07458

Copyright © 2000 by Prentice-Hall, Inc
Upper Saddle River, NJ 07458

Printed in the United States of America
10 9 8 7 6 5 4

ISBN 0-13-087736-0

Prentice Hall International (UK) Limited, *London*
Prentice Hall of Australia Pty. Limited, *Sydney*
Prentice Hall Canada, Inc., *Toronto*
Prentice Hall Hispanoamericana, S.A., *Mexico*
Prentice Hall of India Private Limited, *New Delhi*
Prentice Hall of Japan, Inc., *Tokyo*
Simon & Schuster Asia Pte. Ltd., *Singapore*
Editora Prentice Hall do Brasil Ltda., *Rio de Janeiro*

Contents

Preface

There are countless conflicts that occur in the health-care delivery arenas predicated on cultural misunderstandings. Albeit, many of these misunderstandings are related to universal situations, such as verbal and nonverbal language misunderstandings, the conventions for courtesy, sequencing of interactions, phasing of interactions, objectivity, and so forth; there are, however, countless cultural misunderstandings unique to the delivery of health care. The necessity to provide CulturalCare—professional health care that is culturally sensitive, culturally appropriate, and culturally competent—is essential as we enter the new millennium, and this demands that providers must be able to assess and interpret the given patient's health beliefs and practices. CulturalCare alters the perspective of health-care delivery as it enables the provider to understand, from a cultural perspective, the manifestations of the patient's HEALTH-care beliefs and practices.

This guide presents:

1. **Cultural Conflicts**—a sample of clinical situations in which a provider may encounter situations wherein patients do not adhere to suggested regimens or where other variances in expected patient behavior occur that may be predicated on the patient's ethnocultural heritage;

v

2. **CulturalCare Considerations**—a selection of practical assessment tools, guidelines, and information, the purpose of which is to facilitate communication and caring for the culturally diverse people you will meet in all practice arenas; and

3. **CulturalCare Conclusions**—possible solutions to the scenarios posed in the initial section of this guide.

Each of us comes from a unique cultural heritage, and the health-care system in which we practice may present us with complex cultural dilemmas. As you begin to delve into this topic, apply each of the tools to yourself and then ask the following questions about your personal and professional worlds:

- What is my personal ethnocultural heritage and how deeply do I identify with it?
- What do I know about HEALTH and illness from my own heritage?
- What is my professional heritage and how deeply do I identify with it?
- What have I learned about HEALTH in the contexts of both my personal heritage and the health-care system?

CulturalConflicts

The following scenarios are composite situations that may be encountered in a variety of clinical settings. In order to prevent stereotyping, the heritage of the patient involved in the situation is not given here. Rather, the situations are presented in a generic fashion. The tools for assessment and process are then presented with a subsequent section on selected HEALTH traditions. At the end of the guide, each scenario is revisited and the possible "CulturalCare Conclusions" are presented. They serve to demonstrate how a given situation may, in fact, occur among people from many different ethnocultural backgrounds.

1. A person who is bleeding refuses surgery when they are forced to remove what appears to be a piece of jewelry.
2. A person is admitted to the emergency room with welts and large red circles on their back.
3. A person who is being interviewed refuses to answer questions directly or to look the provider in the eye.
4. An adult immunization clinic is held in a public building and the turnout for the program is minimal.
5. A new mother does not want to hold or see her baby following the delivery.
6. A person on a liquid diet refuses to eat the gelatin.

7. A young patient refuses a blood transfusion and is supported by the family.

8. A patient is given a supply of antibiotics in the emergency room to treat a respiratory infection and leaves the medication behind.

9. A person is acutely ill and does not respond to the questions being asked.

10. A person who is terminally ill is found to have a card hidden under the pillow.

11. The family of a person who died refuses to leave the room.

12. A patient who is 24-hours post–chest surgery does not request pain medication.

CulturalCare Considerations

This section of the guide contains practical guides: Heritage Assessment, CulturalCare Phenomena Affecting HEALTH, CulturalCare Etiquette, HEALTH Traditions Assessment Model, and HEALTH Traditions Assessment Guidelines for the community.

Heritage Assessment Tool

This set of questions can be used to investigate a given patient's or your own ethnic, cultural, and religious heritage. It can help you to perform a heritage assessment to determine how deeply a given person identifies with a particular *tradition*. It is most useful in setting the stage for understanding a person's HEALTH traditions. The greater the number of positive responses, the greater the person's identification with a traditional heritage. The one exception to positive answers is the question about family name change. This question may be answered negatively.

1. Where was your mother born? _____
2. Where was your father born? _____
3. Where were your grandparents born?
   a. Your mother's mother? _____
   b. Your mother's father? _____
   c. Your father's mother? _____
   d. Your father's father? _____
4. How many brothers _____ and sisters _____ do you have?
5. What setting did you grow up in? Urban _____ Rural _____ Suburban _____

6. What country did your parents grow up in?
   Father _____
   Mother _____
7. How old were you when you came to the United States? _____
8. How old were your parents when they came to the United States?
   Mother _____
   Father _____
9. When you were growing up, who lived with you?
   _____

10. Have you maintained contact with
    a. Aunts, uncles, cousins? (1) Yes ____ (2) No ____
    b. Brothers and sisters? (1) Yes ____ (2) No ____
    c. Parents? (1) Yes ____ (2) No ____
    d. Your own children? (1) Yes ____ (2) No ____
11. Did most of your aunts, uncles, cousins live near your home?
    (1) Yes ____ (2) No ____
12. Approximately how often did you visit your family members who lived outside your home?
    (1) Daily ____ (2) Weekly ____ (3) Monthly ____
    (4) Once a year or less ____ (5) Never ____
13. Was your original family name changed?
    (1) Yes ____ (2) No ____
14. What is your religious preference?
    (1) Catholic ____ (2) Jewish ____
    (3) Protestant ____ Denomination _____
    (4) Other ____ (5) None ____
15. Is your spouse the same religion as you?
    (1) Yes ____ (2) No ____
16. Is your spouse the same ethnic background as you?
    (1) Yes ____ (2) No ____
17. What kind of school did you go to?
    (1) Public ____ (2) Private ____ (3) Parochial ____
18. As an adult, do you live in a neighborhood where the neighbors are the same religion and ethnic background as yourself?
    (1) Yes ____ (2) No ____
19. Do you belong to a religious institution?
    (1) Yes ____ (2) No ____

20. Would you describe yourself as an active member?
    (1) Yes ___ (2) No ___
21. How often do you attend your religious institution?
    (1) More than once a week ___ (2) Weekly ___
    (3) Monthly ___ (4) Special holidays only ___
    (5) Never ___
22. Do you practice your religion in your home?
    (1) Yes ___ (2) No ___
    (If yes, please specify)
    (3) Praying ___ (4) Bible reading ___
    (5) Diet ___ (6) Celebrating religious holidays ___
23. Do you prepare foods of your ethnic background?
    (1) Yes ___ (2) No ___
24. Do you participate in ethnic activities?
    (1) Yes ___ (2) No ___
    (If yes, please specify)
    (3) Singing ___ (4) Holiday celebrations ___
    (5) Dancing ___ (6) Festivals ___
    (7) Costumes ___ (8) Other ___
25. Are your friends from the same religious background as you?
    (1) Yes ___ (2) No ___
26. Are your friends from the same ethnic background as you?
    (1) Yes ___ (2) No ___
27. What is your native language? _____
28. Do you speak this language?
    (1) Prefer ___ (2) Occasionally ___ (3) Rarely ___
29. Do you read your native language?
    (1) Yes ___ (2) No ___

CulturalCare Phenomena Affecting HEALTH

Giger and Davidhizar* have identified six cultural phenomena that vary among cultural groups. These are

1. **Environmental control**—The ability of members of a particular cultural group to plan activities that control nature or direct environmental factors. Included are the complex systems of traditional health and illness beliefs, the practice of folk medicine, and the use of traditional healers. These play an extremely important role in the way clients respond to health-related experiences, including the ways in which they define health and illness and seek and use health-care resources and social supports.

2. **Biological variations**—People from one cultural group differ biologically (physically and genetically) from members of other cultural groups:
   a. Body build and structure
   b. Skin color

---

*Giger, J.N. and Davidhizar, R.E. *Transcultural Nursing Assessment and Intervention*, 2nd ed. St. Louis: Mosby, 1995, pp. 19, 43, 61, 89, 113, and 127.

    c. Enzymatic and genetic variations

    d. Susceptibility to disease

    e. Nutritional variations

3. **Social organization**—The family unit, (nuclear, single-parent, or extended family) and the social group organizations (religious or ethnic) with which clients and families may identify.

4. **Communication**—Communication differences are presented in many ways, including language differences, verbal and nonverbal behaviors, and silence.

5. **Space**—Personal space and territoriality involves people's behaviors and attitudes toward the space around themselves and are influenced by culture. The following terms indicate different types of space and relate to acceptable behaviors within these zones:

    a. *Intimate zone:* extends up to 1½ feet.

    b. *Personal distance:* extends from 1½ to 4 feet.

    c. *Social distance:* extends from 4 to 12 feet.

    d. *Public distance:* extends 12 feet or more.

6. **Time orientation**—The viewing of the time in the present, past, or future varies among different cultural groups.

    a. *Future-oriented:* People are concerned with long-range goals and with health-care measures taken in the present to prevent the occurrence of illness in the future.

    b. *Present-oriented:* People are oriented more to the present than the future and may be late for appointments because they are less concerned about planning ahead to be on time.

Cultural Phenomena Affecting Health Care

	African (Black) Americans	Asian/Pacific Islander Americans	American Indians Aleuts, and Eskimos	Hispanic Americans	European (White) Origin Americans
Nations of Origin	West coast (as slaves) of Africa Many African countries West Indian islands Dominican Republic Haiti Jamaica	China, Japan, Hawaii, the Philippines, Vietnam, Asian India, Korea, Samoa, Guam, and the remaining Asian/Pacific islands	200 American Indian nations indigenous to North America Aleuts, and Eskimos in Alaska	Hispanic countries Spain, Cuba, Mexico, Central and South America Puerto Rico	Germany, England, Italy, Ireland, Former Soviet Union, and all other European countries

9

Cultural Phenomena Affecting Health Care (Cont.)

	African (Black) Americans	Asian/Pacific Islander Americans	American Indians Aleuts, and Eskimos	Hispanic Americans	European (White) Origin Americans
Environmental Control	Traditional health and illness beliefs may continue to be observed by "traditional" people	Traditional health and illness beliefs may continue to be observed by "traditional" people	Traditional health and illness beliefs may continue to be observed by "traditional" people Natural and magicoreligious folk medicine tradition Traditional healer: medicine man or woman	Traditional health and illness beliefs may continue to be observed by "traditional" people Folk medicine tradition Traditional healers: *curandero, espiritista, partera, señora*	Primary reliance on "modern, Western" health-care delivery system Remaining traditional health and illness beliefs and practices may be observed Some remaining traditional folk medicine Homeopathic medicine resurgent

Biological Variations				
Sickle cell anemia	Hypertension	Accidents	Diabetes mellitus	Breast cancer
Hypertension	Liver cancer	Heart disease	Parasites	Heart disease
Cancer of the esophagus	Stomach cancer	Cirrhosis of the liver	Coccidioido-mycosis	Diabetes mellitus
Stomach cancer	Coccidioido-mycosis	Diabetes mellitus	Lactose intolerance	Thalassemia
Coccidioido-mycosis	Lactose intolerance			
Lactose intolerance	Thalassemia			

11

Cultural Phenomena Affecting Health Care (Cont.)

	African (Black) Americans	Asian/Pacific Islander Americans	American Indians Aleuts, and Eskimos	Hispanic Americans	European (White) Origin Americans
Social Organization	Family: many single-parent female-headed households Large, extended family networks Strong church affiliations within community Community social organizations	Family: hierarchical structure, loyalty Large, extended family networks Devotion to tradition Many religions, including Taoism, Buddhism, Islam, and Christianity Community social organizations	Extremely family-oriented to both biological and extended families Children are taught to respect traditions Community social organizations	Nuclear families Large, extended family networks *Compadrazzo* (godparents) Strong church affiliations within community Community social organizations	Nuclear families Extended families Judeo-Christian religions Community and social organizations

Communication	National languages Dialect: Pidgin French, Spanish, Creole	National language preference Dialects, written characters Use of silence Nonverbal and contextual cueing	Tribal languages Use of silence and body language	Spanish or Portuguese are the primary languages	National languages Many learned English rapidly as imigrants Verbal, rather than nonverbal
Space	Close personal space	Noncontact people	Space very important and has no boundaries	Tactile relationships: touch, handshakes, embrace Value physical presence	Noncontact people: aloof, distant Southern countries: closer contact and touch
Time Orientation	Present over future	Present	Present	Present	Future over present

Adapted from: Spector, R. "Cultures, Ethnicity, and Nursing," in *Fundamentals of Nursing,* 3rd ed. eds. Potter, P. and Perry, A. (St. Louis: Mosby, 1992), p. 101.

CulturalCare Etiquette

There are countless ways in which the etiquette essential to a satisfactory provider–patient encounter is breached. This table presents an overview of selected situations wherein etiquette can be modified to the needs of a patient.

Cultural Phenomena Affecting Etiquette

Time	Visiting	Inform patient when you are coming
	Being on time	Avoid surprises
		Explain your expectations about time
		Ask patients from other regions and cultures what they expect
	Taboo times	Be familiar with the times and meanings of patient's ethnic and religious holidays
Space	Body language and distances	Know, from many perspectives, cultural and/or religious customs regarding contact and touch with others
Communication	Greetings	Know the proper forms of address for people from a given culture and the ways by which people welcome one another
		Know when touch, such as an embrace or handshake, is expected and when physical contact is prohibited
	Gestures	Gestures do not have universal meaning—what is acceptable to one cultural group is taboo with another
	Smiling	Smiles may be indicative of friendliness to some, taboo to others
	Eye contact	Avoiding eye contact may be a sign of respect

Cultural Phenomena Affecting Etiquette (Cont.)

Social Organization	Holidays	Know what dates are important and why, whether or not to give gifts, what to wear to special events, what the customs and beliefs are
	Special events • Births • Weddings • Funerals	Know how the event is celebrated, meaning of colors used for gifts, expected rituals at home or religious services
Biological Variations	Food customs	Know what can be eaten for certain events, what foods may be eaten together or are forbidden, what and how utensils are used
Environmental Control	Health practices and remedies	Know what the general health traditions are for a given patient and question observations for validity

HEALTH
Traditions
Assessment
Model

People who identify with a traditional ethnocultural heritage may tend to define HEALTH and illness in a holistic way, and have health beliefs and practices that differ from those of the Western, or modern, health-care delivery system.

Imagine holistic HEALTH as a three-dimensional phenomenon that encompasses the following: body (the physical self), mind (feelings, attitudes, and behavior), and spirit (the I who I am).

HEALTH, in the traditional sense, is the state of balance within the body, mind, and spirit, and with the family, community, and the forces of the natural world.

Illness is the opposite.

Many traditional HEALTH beliefs and practices exist today among people who know and live by the traditions of their given ethnocultural heritage.

HEALTH, in this traditional context, has three dimensions each of which has three aspects, making a total of nine interrelated facets.

1. **Maintaining HEALTH**
   a. *Physical*—Are there special clothes one must wear; foods one must eat, not eat, or combinations to avoid; exercises one must do?
   b. *Mental*—Are there special sources of entertainment; games or other ways of concentrating; traditional "rules of behavior"?
   c. *Spiritual*—Are there special religious customs; prayers; meditations?
2. **Protecting HEALTH**
   a. *Physical*—Are there special foods that must be eaten after certain life events, such as childbirth; dietary taboos that must be adhered to; symbolic clothes that must be worn?
   b. *Mental*—Are there special people who must be avoided; rituals for self-protection; familial roles?
   c. *Spiritual*—Are there special religious customs; superstitions; amulets; oils or waters?
3. **Restoring HEALTH**
   a. *Physical*—Are there special folk remedies; liniments; procedures, such as cupping, acupuncture, and moxibustion?
   b. *Mental*—Are there special healers, such as *curanderos,* available; rituals; folk medicines?
   c. *Spiritual*—Are there special rituals and prayers; meditations; healers?

Traditional methods of maintaining, protecting, and restoring HEALTH require the knowledge and understanding of HEALTH-related resources from within a given person's ethnoreligious cultural heritage and community. These methods may be used instead of or along with modern methods of health care. They are not alternative methods of health care in the sense that they are methods that are an integral part of a person's given heritage.

HEALTH
Traditions
Assessment
Guidelines

A given patient's interrelated HEALTH traditions can be assessed in countless ways. The following grids contain suggested questions and are parallel to the nine interrelated facets of HEALTH (the physical, mental, and spiritual aspects of the personal and communal dimensions of maintaining, protecting and restoring HEALTH that are a theme throughout *Cultural Diversity in Health and Illness* and this assessment guide.

Assessment Guide for <u>Personal</u> Methods to Maintain, Protect, and Restore HEALTH

	Physical	Mental	Spiritual
Maintain HEALTH	Are there special clothes you must wear at certain times of the day, week, year? Are there special foods you must eat at certain times? Do you have any dietary restrictions? Are there any foods that you cannot eat?	What do you do for activities, such as reading, sports, games? Do you have hobbies? Do you visit family often? Do you visit friends often?	Do you practice your religions and attend church or other communal activities? Do you pray or meditate? Do you observe religious customs? Do you belong to fraternal organizations?
Protect HEALTH	Are there foods that you cannot eat together? Are there special foods that you must eat? Are there any types of clothing that you are not allowed to wear?	Are there people or situations that you have been taught to avoid? Do you take extraordinary precautions under certain circumstances? Do you take time for yourself?	Do you observe religious customs? Do you wear any amulets or hang them in your home? Do you have any practices, such as always opening the window when you sleep? Do you have any other practices to protect yourself from "harm"?

| Restore HEALTH | What kinds of medicines do you take before you see a doctor or nurse?
Are there herbs that you take?
Are there special treatments that you use? | Do you know of any specific practices your mother or grandmother may use to relax?
Do you know how big problems can be cared for in your community?
Do you drink special teas to help you unwind or relax?
Do you know of any healers? | Do you know of any religious rituals that help to restore health?
Do you meditate?
Did you ever go to a healing service?
Do you know about exorcism? |

Community
HEALTH
Traditions
Assessment
Guidelines

HEALTH traditions come alive the moment one leaves institutional confines and goes into the community. An in-depth community assessment of an ethnoreligious community alerts you to the vast resources that exist within traditional communities and that may be tapped. The following outline serves as a community assessment guide:

Demographic Data

- Total population size of entire city or town
- Breakdown by areas—residential concentrations
- Breakdown by ages
- Other breakdowns
  Education
  Occupations
  Income

- Nations of origin of residents of the location and the target neighborhood

Traditional HEALTH Beliefs

- Definition of HEALTH
- Definition of illness
- Overall HEALTH status

Causes of Illness

- Poor eating habits
- Wrong food combinations
- Viruses, bacteria, other organisms
- Punishment from God
- The evil eye
- Hexes, spells, or envy
- Witchcraft
- Environmental changes
- Exposure to drafts
- Over- or underwork
- Grief and loss

Methods of Maintaining HEALTH

Methods of Protecting HEALTH

Methods of Restoring HEALTH—Home Remedies

Visits and Use of M.D. or Other Health-Care Resources

Health-Care Resources, Such As Neighborhood Health Centers

Anyone Else Within Community Who Looks After People, Such As Traditional Healers

Child-Bearing Beliefs and Practices

Child-Rearing Beliefs and Practices

Rituals and Beliefs Surrounding Death and Dying

Walk through the community and observe the traditional grocery stores, pharmacies, markets, jewelry stores, beauty parlors, morticians, and churches. If possible, visit several places, purchase remedies, eat in a restaurant, and observe services in a church.

Assessment Guide for Communal Methods and Resources for Maintaining, Protecting, and Restoring HEALTH

	Physical	Mental	Spiritual
Maintain HEALTH	Where are people able to purchase special clothing? Where are specific foods purchased? What types of health education are a part of the person's culture and who teaches this information? Where is the information obtained?	What are examples of culture-specific books, games, and other activities for this given client? Where are books, games, and other forms of culture-specific materials obtained? What are culture-specific rules for this patient, such as conversation, eye contact?	Are there resources to meet the patient's identified spiritual needs? How are the people and places accessed?
Protect HEALTH	Where are special clothes obtained? What are some examples of symbolic clothing a person may obtain?	Who within the patient's family and community teaches the cultural rules? Are there rules about avoiding people or places? Are there special activities that must be observed?	Who teaches the spiritual practices? Where can the patient purchase special amulets and other symbolic objects? Are they costly? Are they readily available?

Restore HEALTH		
Where are various remedies purchased? Are people able to grow herbs and other remedies in their own homes? Where are other traditional services obtained? Who are the traditional healers within the patient community and where do they practice?	Who are the traditional people within the community that the person may seek care and advice from? Are there culture-specific activities, such as story telling that may be available to the patient? Where are the ingredients for special "teas" purchased?	Are there traditional healers in the community? Who are they and how are they accessed?

Selected HEALTH Traditions

Nation	Maintain HEALTH	Protect HEALTH	Restore HEALTH
Austria	Soups and sleeping Dress warmly and wear shoes	Use *Schweden-bitter* (herb extract) Promote sweating	Chest cold: Scoop inside of a black radish, fill the cavity with rock candy and bake it. Then drink the contents. Ear aches: Take a white sock and put heated salt inside of it and place it on the ear. Fever: Wrap wet towel around body. Cough: Melt sugar and crystallize with onion juice.
Bangladesh	Eat fruits and rice	Eat a special plant from the rain forest	Use herbs
Bolivia	Sleep, eat, and drink in moderation	Walk	Use cupping to improve circulation
Brazil	Take *Cachaca* Cook and clean all day	Drink herbal teas Eat chicken soup	Drink herbal teas Eat herbs

China	Always clean the floor Use Chinese herbs	Drink ginger tea to prevent the flu	Cough: Scratch the back with a coin Drink herbal teas Diarrhea: Drink a burned rice tea
Colombia	Drink *agua de panela con limon* Eat garlic for general health Eat chicken and rice	Use *botanica* (herbal plants)	Cold: Prepare onions and oil by cooking until pulp is soft, strain, and eat with honey Baby's colic: Prepare star anise tea Nerves: Drink *tilo* Cramps: Cook onion and place on stomach Visit traditional healers

Selected HEALTH Traditions (Cont.)

Nation	Maintain HEALTH	Protect HEALTH	Restore HEALTH
Croatia	Eat organically grown food, goat's milk, fish from the Adriatic Sea	Get plenty of fresh air and exercise	Broken bones: Place a dead animal on the skin Upset stomach: Drink chamomile tea Ear aches: Place hot oil on cotton ball in the ear
Cuba	Drink carrot juice and eat fruits, vegetables, garlic, tea soups, and stews	Dress warmly	Sore throat: Drink olive oil and salt, or a tea of boiled water with lemon rind for 10 minutes then put in cup with regular tea bag and juice of lemon, add honey to sweeten Use pig skins as bandages to cure cuts Visit traditional healers (santero)

Dominican Republic	Use oils or herb teas	Keep the sick inside the house Get a lot of rest Keep out of cold rain	Use plants, oils, and roots for homemade medicines Cover a person with a fever with a heavy blanket for two to three hours until he or she sweats
Ecuador	Eat healthful food; drink teas	Drink teas Wear amulets	Drink teas
England	Take cod liver oil daily	Get lots of fresh air Wrap up warmly Drink brown ale after cleaning a sick room to prevent catching the disease	Fever: Drink mint or chamomile tea Cough and congestion: Put formaldehyde crystals in a plastic bag and place on the chest Mumps: Apply hot mustard poultice Nosebleed: Put a cold key down your back

Selected Health Traditions (Cont.)

Nation	Maintain HEALTH	Protect HEALTH	Restore HEALTH
England (cont.)			General illness: Feed bread cubes in a warm sweet milk (pobs)
Ethiopia	Make sure food is on the table for everyone	Give people water blessed by the spirit (church) to drink	Pray
France	Eat a big lunch with different foods Drink drinks with herbs Drink soup Eat chocolate Take cod liver oil Eat bread and butter Put hot stones under the bed Put iron nails in water	Take cod liver oil (oil of fish liver)	General illness: Drink *Daliborng* water Cuts and bruises: Put castor oil on right away to prevent pain and swelling

Germany	Eat meatball soup, lots of vegetables, and good food Every day before going to bed eat an apple Take cod liver oil Get fresh air, and work hard	Take castor oil daily Dress warmly Wrap salted herring and wear it around your neck Drink boneset tea daily	Colds: Apply mustard plaster Visit neighborhood pow-wow doctors Worms: Eat hot garlic milk with honey Any illness: Eat chicken soup Cold: Place a cut onion next to your bed while sleeping to help breathing
Greece	Eat good food Drink chamomile tea Wear a wool undershirt Never go out of house after bath	Eat 1 tablespoon of honey each day during the cold months to prevent colds Keep warm Wear amulets containing flowers from the Epitafio on Holy Friday Pray to God	Stomach ailments: Drink mountain tea (mint tea with honey) Pray Colds and pneumonia: Use cupping (cotton inserted in a glass and lit with a match and left on the back)

Selected HEALTH Traditions (Cont.)

Nation	Maintain HEALTH	Protect HEALTH	Restore HEALTH
Greece (cont.)			
Haiti	Eat well Eat fresh foods	Drink tea every day made with sorosi to increase appetite	Ear aches: Warm olive oil and place it in the ear Fever: Mix castor oil, alcohol, and shallot. Heat the mixture, rub together in hand, and rub all over the body
India	Eat vegetables Eat healthful foods and exercise	Use black pepper and licorice	Indigestion: Drink cumin water Upset stomach: Drink buttermilk and fenugreek Sore throat: Drink tumeric in hot milk
Ireland	Eat lots of potatoes and cabbage Wear warm clothing Keep clean Get fresh air, and work hard Sleep with the window open a crack	In spring time take nettles (wild), boil them down, and then drink it Eat porridge at night before going to bed Pray	Drink plenty of tea and Guiness (ale) Cold: Eat a whole raw onion and have a shot of whiskey "Wind," (flatulence): Face rear end to the fire

Italy			
Love each other Eat chicken soup Wear and eat garlic Drink a glass of wine a day Wear a camphor bag around the neck Eat fresh fruit and vegetables every day Get lots of sleep	Do not go to bed with wet hair Drink nettle soup to clear the blood Put camphor on a cloth and wear around neck	Children should wear a pouch with raw garlic around neck to keep unhealthy children away "Spring cleaning"—Drink bitter greens boiled in water	Boils and cuts: Wrap hot bread, sugar, soap in linen cloth and place it on the wound to prevent infection Cold or flu: Apply poultices and molasses Fever: Tie onions to wrists or dirty sock around the neck Cold and cough: Put warm to hot red brick wrapped in wool cloth on chest Inhale very hot water with turpentine, or drink boiled wine with apples Get rid of the evil eye or to cast out any evil spirits: Drink cod liver oil Colic: Drink fennel seed tea

Selected HEALTH Traditions (Cont.)

Nation	Maintain HEALTH	Protect HEALTH	Restore HEALTH
Italy (cont.)			Pray to God Upset stomach: Drink water mixed with sugar and bay leaf
Jamaica	Eat a lot of tropical fruits, especially mangoes Get a lot of exercise in the form of chores Take weekly cathartics to wash out the system and drink cerasee tea (each Sunday)	Drink different kinds of herb and bush teas Get plenty of rest Drink whole milk and beef soup, and eat fresh fruit and vegetables	Take medicine in the form of herbal bushes Pray to the Lord for help Back pain: Use a poultice Stomach problems: Drink dandelion and ginger teas
Japan	Children: Every morning (even in winter) massage his or her naked body to keep healthy	Gargle with salt water Sleep well, eat good things, and exercise	Keep body warm with blanket and sleep Cure asthma attacks; yaeto usually burned on upper back and shoulders Upset stomach: Drink green tea

Lithuania	Eat fresh fruits and vegetables Take herbal enemas	Eat good food, get plenty of rest	Apply mustard plasters Colds and stomach aches: Drink brandy
Mexico	Eat eggs and bread Sleep and drink tea	Use herbs and amulets	Use herbs, and visit traditional healers
Netherlands	Practice cleanliness Eat pancakes Eat cooked vegetables	Make sure to get up on the right foot Eat a lot of fruit Eat chicken soup	Headache: Mop the floor with ammonia Eat soft-boiled eggs
Norway	Eat fruit and vegetables	Wear coats and pants	Eat soup and drink hot chocolate
Pakistan	Take lemon in summer to beat the heat Eat chicken soup in the winter	Eat garlic to prevent colds in the winter	Headache: Drink green tea Gas in stomach: Drink ginger

Selected HEALTH Traditions (Cont.)

Nation	Maintain HEALTH	Protect HEALTH	Restore HEALTH
Philippines	Pray Eat healthful food, such as vegetables, meat, chicken, and fruits and have excellent hygiene	Eat pigeon soup After working in the fields, soak feet in salted water Avoid too much sun or rain	Eat chicken soup Painful joints: Pound ginger mix with coconut oil and massage Stomach ache: Toast uncooked rice until brown, add water, mix, and drink the fluid Wounds: Boil guava leaves and drink the fluid, or grind guava leaves and apply to the wound to cure fresh wound faster Take herbal medicines
Poland	Eat chicken soup Tie garlic around neck Eat well (fat) Drink tea with honey or cinnamon Drink tea from Camile tree flowers Practice cleanliness	Dress warmly Eat broth Use herbal tonics Eat garlic	Practice blood letting using leeches Colds: Eat chicken soup, drink hot tea, apply mustard plasters, hot cups, compresses; drink raspberry juice Stomach problems: Drink mint tea

Prussia	Drink herbal teas Eat plantain leaves Drink tea with honey and ground ambgor every day Use feverfew and mint	Wear Yiddish amulets and keep good luck coins	To draw out infection: Apply pitch from pine trees
Romania	Saturday night bath for all children in the same water Eat a balanced diet Eat chicken soup Eat mush and drink fresh milk	Eat garlic daily	Cold or flu: Eat chicken soup To purify blood: Eat garlic Constipation: Eat yogurt and herbs Warts: Apply poultice of chicken skin and mustard
Russia	Eat chicken soup Keep warm Eat lots of vegetables Take cod liver oil Eat raw garlic and onions	Wear garlic bags around the neck Children wear camphor enclosed in a cloth necklace Wear dry socks Keep the feet warm and the head covered	Colds and flu: Use cupping Colds and sore throat: Drink milk with butter; or apply a mustard plaster using dry mustard in a gauze bag and dipping into water and placing on chest

Selected HEALTH Traditions (Cont.)

Nation	Maintain HEALTH	Protect HEALTH	Restore HEALTH
Russia (cont.)			Sore throat: Drink *guggle muggle* (a drink of hot milk, honey [or sugar] and butter) or boil together 1 jigger of wine or brandy, juice of 1 lemon, and 1 tbs. of honey. Drink Stye: Rub eye with wedding ring and spit three times
Slovakia	Eat chicken soup Wash hands Eat cabbage soup Eat prune desserts to keep in balance Eat garlic and sauerkraut (also juice from it) especially in winter Drink herbal teas (chamomile for general health)	Get lots of sleep and exercise Eat garlic Get fresh air Eat a lot of vegetables Keep dry and warm	Cold: Drink tea with honey and lemon Pray (novenas—nine days of praying) Infections: Epson salts in bath water Sore throat: Drink hot milk with squeezed garlic in it plus 2 teaspoons of honey

			Heavy cough, pain in chest: Heat fat in a small pot, apply to a cloth and put on chest until it is covered with a slight film of fat. Cover with plastic (to keep it warm) and blend into towel and try to sleep with it overnight
			Indigestion: Eat garlic soup
Thailand	Take care of children	Eat healthful foods	Use herbs, plants
Turkey	Eat a cup of yogurt a day	Drink hot milk with egg yolk and sugar	Insect bites: Cover with mud mixed with urine
		Keep your feet warm and head cool	Sprains: Apply garlic and raisin poultice to the area
		Don't worry too much	Toothache: Drink brandy
			Minor illness: Boil mint with lemon and drink
			Common cold: Drink linden flower tea

Selected HEALTH Traditions (Cont.)

Nation	Maintain HEALTH	Protect HEALTH	Restore HEALTH
Turkey (cont.)			Blunt injuries (minor): Cover with dough and hammered meat Stye: Apply garlic
Ukraine	Eat chicken soup Drink vodka	Eat healthful food Bundle up in cold weather Drink vodka	Coughs: Use cupping Fever: Apply mustard packs Constipation: Use enemas Cold (stuffy nose): Wrap boiled potatoes in a towel, hold on nose, also mix honey and water as nose drops Drink vodka
Venezuela		Use homeopathic medicine	Upset stomach: Drink hot milk with butter
Vietnam	Eat well Eat soup and drink tea	Use massage Take steambaths Apply tiger oil	Use Chinese medicine

From: Spector, R., Rutberg, C., and Byron, E. Data collected from visitors to "Immigrant Health Traditions" Exhibit, Ellis Island Immigration Museum, May 1994–January 1995.

40

CulturalCare Guide*

The following guidelines will help you understand your patients better and allow you to provide the needed help.

Preparing

- Understand your own cultural values and biases.
- Acquire basic knowledge of cultural values, HEALTH beliefs and practices for the client groups you serve.
- Be respectful of, interested in, and understanding of other cultures without being judgmental.

Enhancing Communication

- Determine the patient's level of fluency in English and arrange for an interpreter, if needed.
- Ask how the patient prefers to be addressed.
- Allow the patient to choose seating for comfortable personal space and eye contact.
- Avoid body language that may be offensive or misunderstood.

---

*From: Schilling, B. and Brannon, E. Cross-Cultural Counseling—A Guide for Nutrition and Health Counselors. Alexandria, VA: (United States Department of Agriculture, United States Department of Health and Human Services, Nutrition and Technical Services Division, September, 1986), p. 19. Reprinted with permission.

- Speak directly to the patient, whether an interpreter is present or not.
- Choose a speech rate and style that promotes understanding and demonstrates respect for the patient.
- Avoid slang, technical jargon, and complex sentences.
- Use open-ended questions or questions phrased in several ways to obtain information.
- Determine the patient's reading ability before using written materials in the teaching process. If patient cannot read English, translate materials.

Promoting Positive Change

- Build on cultural practices, reinforcing those that are positive, and promoting change only in those that are harmful.
- Check for patient understanding and acceptance of recommendations.
- *Remember:* Not all seeds of knowledge fall into a fertile environment to produce change. Of those that do, some will take years to germinate. Be patient and provide care in a culturally appropriate environment to promote positive health behavior.

CulturalCare Conclusions

Each of the cases presented in the beginning of this guide book can be understood if viewed through a lens of CulturalCare. Initially, the patient in each scene must be assessed with the Heritage Assessment tool. Once the given patient's ethnocultural history is learned and the degree to which this person identifies with the given tradition detected, emphasis must be placed on discovering the role that the given heritage plays in the situation. Each situation has specific reasons for occurring within a cultural context. The text, *Cultural Diversity in Health and Illness*, 5th ed., provides a much deeper theoretical background relevant to each of the situations. A summary is presented here.

1. A person who is bleeding refuses surgery when they are forced to remove what appears to be a piece of jewelry.

   This person may be from an ethnocultural tradition where amulets are worn and the removal of the amulet may precede certain death. The amulet is believed to protect the person from external evils and the person may be reluctant to remove it for this reason. The person may be from an African, Hispanic, Asian, or European heritage.

2. A person is admitted to the emergency room with welts and large red circles on their back.

> The person may come from an ethnocultural tradition where coining or cupping are used to treat many maladies, especially respiratory infections. These traditional practices include people from Asian and Eastern European heritages.

3. A person who is being interviewed refuses to answer questions directly or to look the provider in the eye.

> The person may come from an ethnocultural tradition that places a taboo on interviews where the recording of answers is taboo and/or eye contact with strangers is prohibited. The heritages may include, but are not limited to, American Indian, African American, and Moslem.

4. An adult immunization clinic is held in a public building and the turnout for the program is minimal.

> The person may come from an ethnocultural tradition wherein it is believed that immunization is not necessary for adults, especially the elderly. Many believe that since they were not immunized as children, it is not necessary now. Others believe that diet, amulets, and other practices serve to protect their HEALTH. This phenomena may be observed among people from all heritages.

5. A new mother does not want to hold or see her baby following the delivery.

> The mother may come from an ethnocultural tradition where she has been socialized to believe that the baby must not be bonded with until it is a certain age, as it is vulnerable to outside evil forces. Many rituals of a religious or ethnocultural nature must be observed until the baby is seen to be free from a state of taboo and then bonding is permissible. This may be observed among people from Middle Eastern countries. Also, it may be observed that the mother, or grandmother, may place a red ribbon on the baby.

6. A person on a liquid diet refuses to eat the gelatin.

> The person may come from an ethnocultural tradition that prohibits the eating of pig and/or animal

products and gelatin is made from pig bones, unless specified as "kosher." Jews and Muslims who follow the kosher diet may reject this food.

7. A young patient refuses a blood transfusion and is supported by the family.

   The person may come from an ethnocultural tradition that prohibits the use of blood. This is especially seen when caring for Jehovah's Witnesses, but other religions also prohibit the use of blood.

8. A patient is given a supply of antibiotics in the emergency room to treat a respiratory infection and leaves the medication behind.

   The person may come from an ethnocultural tradition that rejects the use of Western medications. The person may elect to use traditional medications and seek the services of a traditional herbalist. This is observed among Hispanics and Asian Americans.

9. A person is acutely ill and does not respond to the questions being asked.

   The person may come from an ethnocultural tradition that views the answering of direct questions to be taboo. The given person may prefer to answer questions that are asked indirectly and where metaphors are used as statements. This practice is found among American Indians.

10. A person who is terminally ill is found to have a card hidden under the pillow.

    The person may come from an ethnocultural tradition that holds beliefs in healing. A patient I once cared for had hidden a prayer card for St. Peregrine, the patron saint of cancer sufferers, under her pillow and stated that she felt that this was more comforting than any words someone could offer her.

11. The family of a person who died refuses to leave the room.

    The family of the recently deceased person may come from an ethnocultural tradition that believes that the soul of the person must be protected and the body must be ritually cared for by members of the family and/or religious community.

12. A patient who is 24-hours post–chest surgery does not request pain medication.

> The person may come from an ethnocultural tradition that believe in "saving face" and that to complain of pain is taboo. This belief is particularly common among Chinese people.

Needless to say, even with these brief scenarios and explanations there is the danger of stereotyping. However, the situations are real—they occurred within the scope of my own practice and experiences. When situations such as these occur, the most important aspect of care is to have the "cultural" antenna sharp and to question the patient, the family, and/or community people to determine the ethos of the patient's cultural beliefs and practices. In this way, a proper way can be found to avoid harming the patient and holding respect for the patient's cultural traditions.

Selected CulturalCare Terms

CulturalCare—a concept that describes professional health care that is culturally sensitive, culturally appropriate, and culturally competent.

Culturally appropriate—implies that the health-care provider applies the underlying background knowledge that must be possessed to provide a given patient with the best possible health care.

Culturally competent—implies that within the delivered care the health-care provider understands and attends to the total context of the patient's situation including awareness of immigration, stress factors, and cultural differences.

Culturally sensitive—implies that the health-care providers possess some basic knowledge of and constructive attitudes towards the diverse cultural groups found in the setting in which they are practicing.

Emerging Majority—People of color—Black; Asian or Pacific Islander; American Indian, Eskimo, or Aleut; and Hispanic origin, who are expected to comprise a majority of the American population by the year 2020.

HEALTH—the balance of the person, both within one's being—physical, mental, and spiritual—and in the outside environment—natural, familial and communal, and metaphysical.

HEALTH maintenance—the traditional beliefs and practices, such as daily health-related activities, diet, exercise, rest, and clothing, used to maintain HEALTH.

HEALTH protection—the traditional beliefs and practices about what should be done on special occasions or on an ongoing basis for HEALTH protection, such as food taboos and wearing amulets.

HEALTH restoration—the traditional beliefs and practices concerning the activities, such as the use of folk remedies and healers, that must be used to restore HEALTH.

Sample Grid for Cultural Health Assessment

	Physical	Mental	Spiritual
Maintain HEALTH			
Protect HEALTH			
Restore HEALTH			